YOUR KNOWLEDGE HAS VALUE

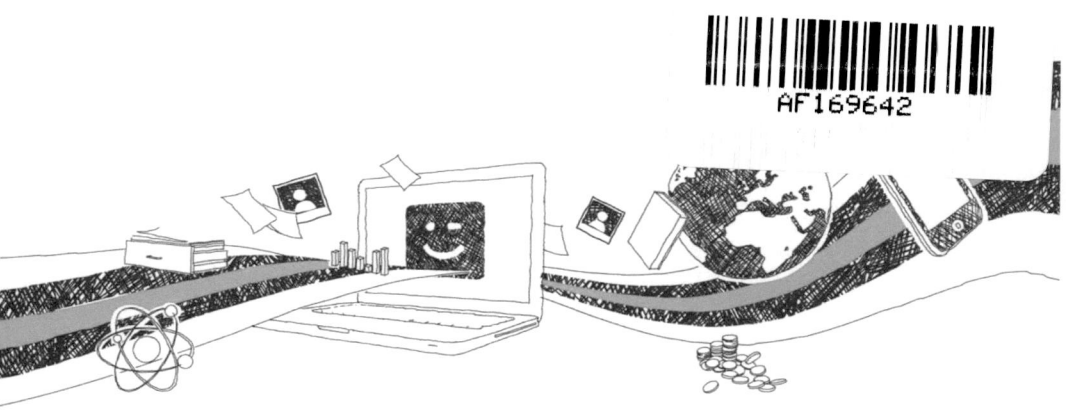

- We will publish your bachelor's and master's thesis, essays and papers

- Your own eBook and book - sold worldwide in all relevant shops

- Earn money with each sale

Upload your text at www.GRIN.com
and publish for free

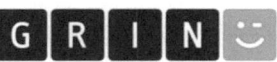

Bibliographic information published by the German National Library:

The German National Library lists this publication in the National Bibliography; detailed bibliographic data are available on the Internet at http://dnb.dnb.de .

This book is copyright material and must not be copied, reproduced, transferred, distributed, leased, licensed or publicly performed or used in any way except as specifically permitted in writing by the publishers, as allowed under the terms and conditions under which it was purchased or as strictly permitted by applicable copyright law. Any unauthorized distribution or use of this text may be a direct infringement of the author s and publisher s rights and those responsible may be liable in law accordingly.

Imprint:

Copyright © 2016 GRIN Verlag, Open Publishing GmbH
Print and binding: Books on Demand GmbH, Norderstedt Germany
ISBN: 9783668429024

This book at GRIN:

http://www.grin.com/en/e-book/349897/drug-abuse-withstanding-the-changing-needs-of-addiction

Robert Kosiba

Drug Abuse. Withstanding the Changing Needs of Addiction

GRIN Publishing

GRIN - Your knowledge has value

Since its foundation in 1998, GRIN has specialized in publishing academic texts by students, college teachers and other academics as e-book and printed book. The website www.grin.com is an ideal platform for presenting term papers, final papers, scientific essays, dissertations and specialist books.

Visit us on the internet:

http://www.grin.com/

http://www.facebook.com/grincom

http://www.twitter.com/grin_com

Introduction 2

Healthcare Addiction needs of the case mothers getting addicted to the prescription pills. 2

What makes people change to addictive nurture based on the mothers getting addicted to prescription pills? 3

The best treatment for healthcare providers when handling cases of addiction 4

How addiction can lead to imprisonment 5

Steps on coping with addictive personality and diseases within the clinical /inmate population 6

Opioid addiction 7

The role of providers in managing the addiction issue 8

Conclusion 8

References 9

Introduction

A lot of people do not understand which individual can be addicted to drugs or how drugs can change one's thinking system to an extent where he/she become a substance abuse person. Many researchers view these two occurrences as either social problem or just weak morals in an individual's life. However, one common standard and belief amongst all the researchers is that drug addict can stop abusing drugs and possibly avert addiction only if they decide to change their overall behaviors and will power

In this research, therefore, our primary concern will be to examine health addiction needs, discuss why people change from just regular drug users to a drug addict especially mothers becoming addicted to the prescription pills. The study also examines the best treatment for health care providers handling cases of addiction in health facilities; it also highlighted how these habits could lead to imprisonment. Finally, the paper will also look into steps on coping with addictive personality and diseases within the clinical /inmate population plus what an Opioid addiction is; besides it will also look into the role of providers in managing the dependency issue.

Healthcare Addiction needs of the case mothers getting addicted to the prescription pills.

Prescription medicine is much easier to access than they use to be before. It is this kind of accessibility that has made these drugs to be more of destructive to young families. However for these mothers much as the doctor recommended dose they tend to spiral into out of control addiction.

Addiction to prescription pill starts when the body cannot function with normality, mothers develop a need for these pills before doing anything, this result in none ending the pain, especially back pain. The pain becomes too chronic and can last for months without going away hence making them develop the need to use pain relievers' pills so that the pain can ease.

Additionally, the need for the addiction of the drugs especially the prescription pills comes as result of the need of confident and control amongst mothers. Even though the aim of these pills is for therapeutic purposes, some women go a notch further by using them to enhance their level of confidence as well as their ability to control their feeling. If by change the prescription pills run out they have to go back the doctors to convince them so that she can get the refill.

Though any drugs whether tablet or any other over the counter drugs, one requirement is that the patient needs to be very opened to her doctor regarding the necessity of the medicine. However, this case is not so with several women, some prefer, lying and even changing the physicians whom they prefer to give them the pills, it this kind of cheat which leads to them developing high addiction rate amongst mothers using these pills.

What makes people change to addictive nurture based on the mothers getting addicted to prescription pills?

Prescription drugs abuse refer to the process with which patients use the medication without proper prescription by medical professional thus in turn creating element of substance (Anton, 2010)

In the case of mothers getting addicted to prescription pills which they frequently use, factors such as availability of the medicines attributed to this since most of these drugs do not require the mothers to give a lot of explanations as to why they need to use them. Most women take the opportunity to frequently use them which in turn leads to change in addictive nurture. Besides the rate at which these pills are in circulation is alarming, these drugs are easily available over the counters hence making most people to lay their hand on them. Hence their long-term effects is addictiveness to their use

Demand for the drugs can also explain the increase in addictive nurture amongst most women goes to the doctors while in pain, and they expect to walk out with at least prescription. As noted by the chief medical officer at the Hazelden medical facility, doctors after studying the demand for this painkillers, they see it less time to consume just to write the patient prescription than turning them away. It is this attitude by medical practitioners which leave patients to feel happier and also feel relief without considering the long term effect these will cause. Besides the higher amount of drugs they receive will make them be more dependency on them hence creating the addictive nurture towards using them.

Finally, the huge supply of these pills in the market also plays a lead role in increasing the addictive nurture amongst substance abuse patients. The supply makes it far much simpler for mothers to lay their hands on these pills. According to study conducted by Center for Disease Control and Prevention in collaboration with Oak Ridge Institute for Science and Education, it noted that close to 29% of women usually borrow and share prescription drugs this indeed increases the addictive nurture to mothers while using these pills(CDC, n.d, 2011)

The best treatment for healthcare providers when handling cases of addiction

Even though addiction to these drugs originated from environmental, behavioral, past exposure to these drugs, genetically alteration as well as the neurochemical changes in the brain which are mainly as result of long time exposure(Kreek et al., 2012). A proper treatment with at most accuracy should be channeled to help solve this; health providers should put their efforts in trying to address the above areas where these drug abuses mostly originate.

The best and the most appropriate mode which provider can help in managing most of the addiction is to try to stop the stigmatization amongst the patients. According to the study conducted by Howard and Chung, society tends to stigmatize addiction; this view usually influences nurses thinking ways towards the patient with addiction (Howard and Chung, 2000). However, with the new study, health care providers who develop positive attitude the addict do provide an excellent therapeutic medication to the patients who in turn help them to fully recover (Cleary, Hunt, Malins, Matheson, and Escott 2009).

Motivation is another form of treatment which the health provider can offer. As noted by Livingston and others, motivational interviewing is one of the most efficient remedies to the drug addicts; it usually helps the user to reduce the rate of drug use(Livingston, Milne, Fang, & Amari, 2012). Together with frequent communication with the counselor, the addict can quickly help to identify her goals for future hence making them see the need for reducing drug use.

How addiction can lead to imprisonment

Drug addiction usually alters the state of the mind of the person using the drug; they cannot think positive and straight since their brain has changed. In the case of women, substance abuse can lead one in committing illegal abortion which is punishable by law. According to the study in 2013 in the Journal of Health, Politics, Policy and Law, it noted that close to 413 arrests had been carried out against women for their conduct while pregnant (Meyer et. al, 2007).

Another way on how drug and substance abuse can lead to imprisonment, it that after certain use of the medicine that the state of one's mind change some people engage in an act such as stealing or even becoming violence hence making them face the full force of the law.

Additionally, apart from acquiring drugs by deceit, it is also a crime to use the drug in the wrong way. According to James Forman Junior who is a law professor at Yale University, of late close to 99% of people jailed due to drug-related case are either in possession of them or just applied wrong use of the drugs

In cases of pregnant mothers using prescription pills in a way that is not authorized by the medical practitioner, if the baby dies as a result of the prescription abuse, according to Oklahoma law, the mother can easily be charged by the first degree of murder. The argument is that by the fact that the mother was abused the drug while pregnant, it was a clear indication that the sole aim was to harm the unborn child.

Steps on coping with addictive personality and diseases within the clinical /inmate population

Even though similarities between the two on how to cope up with addictive personality within the general people and those under the criminal system. One common thing is how to address the psychological problems which result from the addiction. The step should be in such a way that it addresses interpersonal difficulties with family, sustaining the relationship as well as management of emotional and psychological problems.

One of the key steps is to develop a cognitive behavioral method which involves, thinking for a change (Jone et al., 2008). According to this method, it will help the addict to have a cognitive self-change where one learns how to examine their thinking as well as their feelings.

Besides, the method will help one to acknowledge social skills development where an addict can easily explore the entire available channel to address the anti-social/ criminal behaviors.

Enhancing problem-solving skill development helps the addictive drug inmate to learn how to use their acquired skills during their time in jail so us to help them avoid engaging in the further use of the drug which can get them jailed again.

Opioid addiction

Opioids are medication design to relieve pain. They reduce the overall intensity of pain signal reaching the brain especially in areas where emotions are high thus reducing the painful stimulus. However, Opioids addiction amongst pregnant women is on the rise, according to the National Survey on Drugs Use and Health estimate that close to 4.4% are reported to be using illicit heroin or analgesics in the last 30 days(Substance Abuse and Mental Health Services Administration,2011). Also close to 1% of pregnant women do use the none prescribe the use of opioids containing pain medication (Azadi &Dildy, 2008). Opioids addiction usually occurs when most women start to constant use prescription of Opioid analgesic or just heroin. Much as most Opioid drugs are mainly for easing the pain, the initial onset or euphoria develop through the utilization of this medication varies especially on how the drug was taken and formulated. Though opioids tend to bind the opioid receptors in the brain leading to the production of pleasurable sensation, it can also lead into depressing respiration which in turn can create respiratory arrest or even death to the addicts. As noted in the other studies, opioids addiction do usually associate with a compulsive drug seeking characteristics, physical dependence as well as tolerance which usually have a long-term effect characterized by the need for ever higher dose(NIDA, n.d, 2014).

The role of providers in managing the addiction issue

Professionals play key roles in managing the addiction issues, according to the study conducted by NIDA, professionals play a core role in screening, provision of brief intervention, referring to the addict for treatment where necessary and lastly provision of ongoing monitoring and follow-up(NIDA, n.d, 2014). From the study, screening and brief intervention which form the core base of the role of the providers was view as not to be labeled as time-consuming since instead they quickly integrate into general medical settings

Conclusion

From the above findings, much as addiction start as a self-desire to help individual fulfill the pleasure, the impact created by this abuse of substance are far much severe since it affects everyone in the society. Besides, it is this vast effect which makes addiction which calls for all people to join to help change the overall need of addiction

References

Anton, R.(2010).Drug abuse is a disease of the human brain: With Focus Focus on alcohol. *Journal of Law, Medicine, and Ethics.* 38(4):735–744. [PubMed]

Azadi, A.& Dildy, G. (2008). Universal screening for substance abuse at the time of parturition. *Am J Obstet Gynecol* ;198:e30–2. [PubMed]

Centers for Disease Control and Prevention (CDC).(2011). The Hepatitis C FAQs for health professionals.

Cleary M, Malins, G. Matheson S, Hunt, G. (2009). Drug and alcohol education for consumer workers and caregivers: A pilot project on the assessment of attitudes toward people with mental illness and addiction to substance use. *Archives of Psychiatric Nursing.* ;23(2):104–110. [PubMed]

Howard M., Chung S.(2000). Nurses' attitudes towards substance abuse people. *Surveys. Substance Use & Misuse.* ;35(3):347–365.

Jones, H., Johnson, E., O'Grady, K., Jasinski, D., Tuten, M., Milio, L.(2008) Dosing adjustments in postpartum patients maintained on buprenorphine or methadone. *J Addict Med* .2:103–7.

Kreek, M., Levran, O., Reed, B., Schlussman, S., Zhou, Y., &Butelman, R.(2012). Opiate addiction and cocaine addiction: Underlying molecular neurobiology and genetics. The *Journal of Clinical Investigation.* 122(10):3387.

Livingston, J., Fang, M., Amari, E., & Milne, T.,(2012) The effectiveness of interventions in reducing stigma related issue against drug abuse patient: *A systematic review.*

Meyer, M., Benvenuto, A., Wagner, K., Plante, D., &Howard, D.(2007). The Intrapartum and postpartum analgesia for women maintained on methadone during pregnancy. *Obstet Gynecol*. 110:261–6. [PubMed] [Obstetrics & Gynecology]

National Institute on Drug Abuse. (2014). Drug Facts: Heroin. Bethesda, MD: *National Institute on Drug Abuse*. Available at http://www.drugabuse.gov/publications/drugfacts/heroin.

Substance Abuse and Mental Health Services Administration.(n.d) (2011). The Results from the 2010 Drug Use and Health National Survey and the summary of national findings.

YOUR KNOWLEDGE HAS VALUE

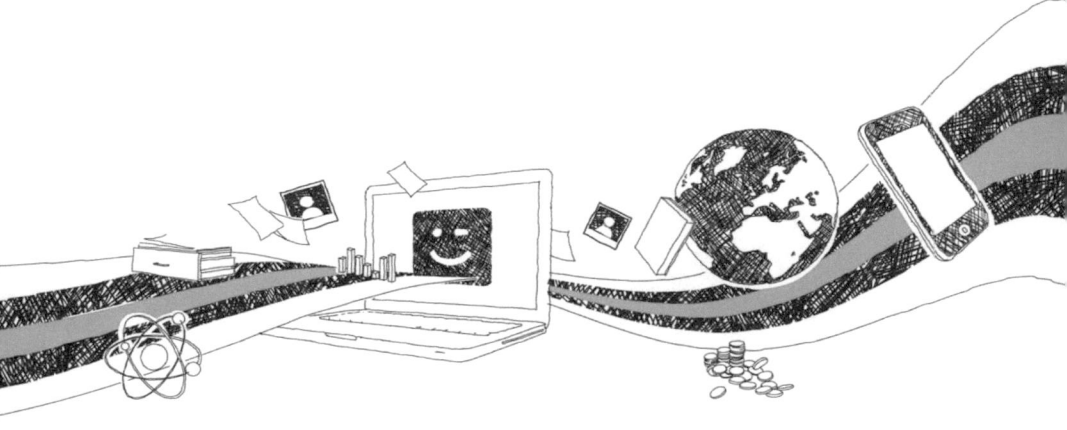

- We will publish your bachelor's and master's thesis, essays and papers

- Your own eBook and book - sold worldwide in all relevant shops

- Earn money with each sale

Upload your text at www.GRIN.com
and publish for free

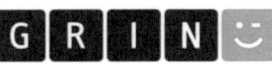